SAR SHALOM
DYNASTY

Amber Rae Johnson Diaz

DEDICATION

I'd like to dedicate my book to two very important people to me. Arlin Llido "My superwoman" for being the example of courage and success in healthcare. Arlin has been there for me mentally , physically and emotionally and I'm grateful for her life and giving me hope. Dr. Torey Troggio has been the key factor in my healing and successfully living out my best life. I'd also like to acknowledge my family and loved ones for being my support system

ABOUT THE AUTHOR

My book is based on my journey and my road to healing—How spirituality and BDSM helped me to heal and overcome some of the most difficult times in life. How due to rejection and difficult times, I had given up on God. Until I met "A Special Friend," and he changed my perspective on life to a positive one, and I was able to let go of my past to walk into my future. For things that seemed impossible or too scary, he made them easy, and I'm grateful to have a friend like him.

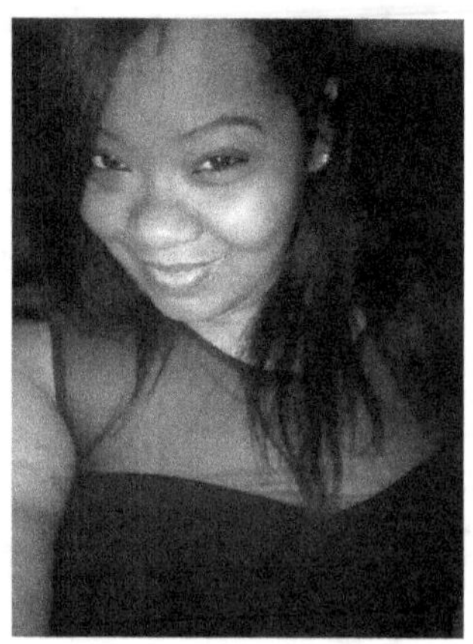

CONTENTS

PREFACE

Decoding Sar Shalom Dynasty

Why this book? Why this title? These are likely the first questions on your mind.

I chose this title to spark curiosity and to reflect the essence of my healing journey. It's more than words on a cover. It's an invitation to explore your own resilience, vulnerability, and healing. Each word carries weight, shaped by years of struggles and revelations.

I chose the Sar Shalom Dynasty as the title of my book. I wanted to convey the idea of peace and strength passed down through generations, much like a lineage of resilience.

The term Sar Shalom means "Prince of Peace"—a symbol of inner calm within life's chaos. This book is my way of sharing the peace I've found within, hoping it reaches you and empowers you in your own journey.

This book is born from personal experience.

It's not just a collection of ideas but a testament to overcoming challenges, accepting imperfections, and rediscovering the strength within. Its purpose is simple: to guide you toward understanding your unique power and using it to transform your life.

You might wonder what to expect from these pages. To start, expect honesty.

This book doesn't sugarcoat life's hardships, nor does it offer quick fixes. Instead, it offers a process: a way to navigate the complexities of life, grow through struggles, and find peace.

Expect tools, not rules.

You'll discover strategies for self-awareness, emotional balance, and self-care.

These aren't rigid instructions but adaptable ideas meant to fit your journey.

Above all, expect connection. This book was written with the hope that you'll see yourself in its stories.

Whether you're battling mental health challenges, seeking purpose, or simply curious about self-discovery, there's something here for you.

This book is more than a guide. It's a conversation. A conversation about healing in ways you never thought possible, practicing spirituality, and reclaiming the strength of self-care.

It's about facing life's obstacles head-on and finding the light that's been there all along.

My stories aren't a guide; they're a mirror that reflects what's possible when you dare to grow.

Turn these pages with an open heart.

You're not alone.

Let's walk this path together.

I

Superpowers We Never Knew We Possessed

"Human emotions are as deep as the ocean, as real as God—stemming from experiences disguised as weaknesses."

- Amber Rae Johnson Diaz

We humans are complex creatures. Our emotions deep. Our thoughts wild. Our actions? Unpredictable. All this contributes to the stringing of stories that are unique in their nature. While the struggles of two individuals may seem the same, deeper into the matter, everything is different. This 'uniqueness' is what fills this world with countless different stories, growing from different roots and curating experiences that allow people to learn, adapt, and make it far in life.

The question, however, that stands is: what is that one thing that connects us and makes us all humans?

We're all blessed with superpowers—powers that most of us are unaware of, powers that can lead us out of our struggles, powers that can direct us to a path of sustainability and success in life.

Resilience. Vulnerability.

Resilience is an innate characteristic—that shows up when you least expect it—which people believe is more of a personality trait. Vulnerability is a state of your mind, body, and soul, which people tend to look upon as a weakness. Humans fail to realize that these two elements are, at their core, our most powerful strengths. Resilience is not something you can learn; rather, it is a characteristic that is embedded deep within you. When you find the courage to tackle the challenges in life, you are being resilient in the face of adversities.

These two are elements that humans need to acclimatize themselves with to transition into their best selves.

Life pushes you down and throws your way situations that at first seem impossible to get out of. It piles on your adversities that may feel like a dead end. Yet, you get back on your feet. It may take you a few days, weeks, months, or even years—but you do get back up. This is human nature.

And this is what we call resilience.

During these difficult times, where you're being resilient, you find yourself at your lowest. You feel everything too deeply. Everything around you feels like it's crushing you. There's a whole lot of rubble and debris piling up on you—you find yourself at the edge, a little more, and you will give up. At this lowest point, you become sensitive to your surroundings. The negative emotions—anger, sadness, anxiety—heighten.

This is your vulnerable state.

While these two may come across as entirely different concepts, from a broader perspective, they are more connected than we know. When surrounded by uncertainties, with hopelessness creeping in, we find ourselves in vulnerable states, pushing us to stand tall in the face of these challenges. These two concepts have the same roots, originating from the same turmoil, grief, and uncertainty.

These two act as tools that lead us to a path toward the light at the end of the tunnel. Together, these can help us come out of even the most difficult situations with their powerful balance. Where vulnerability is what allows us to acknowledge and embrace the pain we are experiencing, resilience is what empowers us to heal from that pain and rise above it. With this power combination, we grow into compassionate and strong individuals.

This all may seem theoretical. Easier said than done, right?

*****

Welcome to my world—the world of Amber Rae Johnson Diaz—I love to refer to myself as the 'Black Diamond.' Working as a Licensed Vocational Nurse for almost two decades, I am at a stage in life where I have found the three Cs: comfort, composure, and calm. From being someone stuck in a rut of mental illnesses and trauma, I have become a dreamer, a pursuer, a strong individual with an aim as high as mountains. I dream to be a nurse consultant and train and educate others like me to become prodigies.

Was I born like this? No.

Was I destined for this? Yes.

These are two very critical aspects of our lives. None of us are born in ideal states. None of us enter the world with passions and dreams. We breathe, we live, we survive—that is how we become individuals who develop an understanding of this world and ourselves. We are not born warriors; we transition into them thanks to our life experiences. But we are born with destinies to fulfill. The traits and tools needed to fulfill our destiny are what we acquire along the way.

By the tools and traits, I mean the innate characteristics and our state of body, mind, and soul: resilience and vulnerability.

I discovered these powers within me the hard way. But better late than never, right?

The wisdom I possess today isn't intrinsic; I had to sit with my ugliest and the darkest thoughts to be here. It took me significant resilience to accept certain turning points. Initially and for many years after, it seemed uncomfortable. With time, in difficult times and scenarios, I made a habit of maintaining calm and listening to understand, not retaliate.

I learned the difference between pain and suffering; while pain is natural, suffering is an active choice. I decided for myself to never suffer. I found things that made my mind feel at ease. One significant part of it was my career path, which added value to my opinions. I have always been passionate about being a nurse. In the near future, hopefully, I also plan on opening learning centers for children. I wish to create a place implementing strategies where kids are eager to dive into wisdom and not consider knowledge a burden. The sole thought of making a noteworthy impact in multiple lives gets my motor running. I've learned that I must ensure that my logic and emotions get along with each other to produce an outcome. They shouldn't be battling against one another; if anything, they should be able to complement each other. Making a career in nursing helped me achieve that goal. I believe that in this era of growing negativity, where most individuals are hell-bent on putting each other down, one person could bring about a significant change.

While I was growing up, all I craved was a normal family that supported one another, but living with five siblings, a father who was least bothered with what we were doing, and a mother who never cared enough to understand, I found myself lost in darkness. As years went by, I grew up to be bitter towards my mom. The underlying reason for this was that she never attempted to care for me the way a child needs. She disregarded my unstable mental health and called me 'lazy' for having it. I particularly did not fancy how she prioritized her convenience, costing further and severe mental disability for me. As for my dad, he was never invested in our lives. My relationship with my mother existed along the lines of resentments mostly initiated by my side. The underlying reason for the negativity instilled in me was the encounters I had when men decided to begin a physical relationship with me without my consent and at my vulnerable age. Dealing with sexual abuse was a big deal in itself, but what left me hopeless was my mom's insensitive reaction to it. I had glimpses of my childhood at several instances when different men molested me. Due to this, I couldn't dare to blink an eye for many years. Whenever I lost consciousness, images from those horrifying experiences would appear in front of my eyes, making it impossible for me to live with myself.

They say paranoia is a disease; I say you haven't experienced life being a girl. Those delusions we hear on the internet and television can be extremely real. I don't remember a time in my life before this when I felt safe in my skin. The world indulged in chaos, and my heart wanted to feel free. Dealing with this kind of experience was the worst thing that happened; it shattered my self-esteem, but little did I know what was coming ahead would make it impossible for me to breathe. When I reached the age of seventeen, my stepfather laid his hands on me. I couldn't stay quiet even if I wanted to, considering he was my mom's husband, so I decided to be vocal about it, at least to my mom. Soon after admitting it to her, she made me regret it. I was already in a vulnerable situation, mentally. There were times when I found myself losing breath; I could die in that moment, or at least that's how it felt. I didn't have anything to move forward with after my mom gave the worst possible reaction anyone could have ever shown. Instead of holding her husband accountable, she blamed me for being the victim. It looked to me as if my life had come to an end, that there was no moving on from this. I had completely given up hope and the will to survive. I was already dead inside; it was just the physical body that needed a rest that lasted forever. I still remember spiraling in my thoughts; I only wondered how everything had fallen apart in a jiff. At this point, I was the most distant with the practices of faith as well because what was supposed to be my safe space also held me accountable for the ill happened to me.

Moving forward, even my teenage dating years were pretty rough; I made mistakes I couldn't undo. I came out as bisexual during my early teens, so I had a couple of experiences with both genders. I didn't possess clarity about the expectations I had from my partner. I had a daughter at the age of twenty-four out of wedlock.

It's safe to say that I've had a fair share of troubles in almost all aspects of my life, perhaps because of my natural ability to learn things the hard way. I've had interactions with severe mental illnesses that, at one point, made me feel like I was on my deathbed. But life is unpredictable; it has its way of uncovering its realities through some gut-wrenching moments before revealing the hope of light.

But what do you have to do with all this that I have suffered from throughout my life?

There's so much that you can learn from my experiences.

Being neglected by the only people you can rely on, your parents, being molested by men of your father's age, being pushed into the gender dilemma at a young age, being confused about your own preferences, and suffering through mental illnesses.

Despite this, despite all the hardships I endured, today I am at a stage in life where I dream—dream big. Producing prodigies with my training center and opening a spa resort where people like me can come in, relax, and unwind. The long journey that I have traveled has led me to realize how important of a role my resilience and vulnerability played. If I lacked the courage to stand tall against these hardships and hadn't reached the most vulnerable state, I wouldn't be here, dreaming of a beautiful life.

My past tells me there is nothing in this universe I can't get; regardless of how rough it might get, I'll walk myself to the absolute end of it.

Even though my life was difficult, there were instances that powered my resilience and became a catalyst in my healing journey. I found what I call accountability partners along the way; some helped me keep my mental state in check, while others introduced me to the most unconventional ways of healing. I was able to connect with my innermost desires. Being bisexual, I've dated quite a few women. By building a dynamic that relies on control and trust, my partners made me feel comfortable in my skin and let me express my true self. I learned that the hate that I projected externally was, in fact, internal.

With resilience comes acceptance, and vulnerability offers you the space you need to grow into your best self.

My experiences and emotions have weaved a story that offers people stuck in life's difficult situations to realize the superpowers that we possess. The emotions that we tend to look upon as weaknesses are indeed treasurable, paving for us a path that takes us closer to that 'light' at the end of the tunnel that everyone's talking about.

II

Roadblocks Or A Step Forward To A Beautiful Life?

"Do you know the steps that you need to climb to build a beautiful life are not your achievements but rather your adversities, failures, heartbreaks, and trauma?"

\-   Amber Rae Johnson Diaz

There's always a different way to look at things driven by unique perspectives and mindsets. While this is a fact, there's a disturbing trend that's taking over, and it's about adopting the perspectives held by the majority. When the world can benefit from different perspectives, thought processes, and approaches, people today fear uniqueness as it is now met with much criticism. This leads to the prevalence of habits, thoughts, and ideas that are plagued with toxicity and negativity.

As there's no one-size-fits-all to live life, there's no one mindset that fits all.

This is what brings me to explore how, unfortunately, the majority of the world's population today looks upon their weaknesses and failures as roadblocks, something that is hindering their success. These people fail to realize the true power of their emotions. If channeled and managed the right way, even the most vulnerable of feelings can turn into their superpowers.

The worst thing about this situation is that we, as humans, believe we're not in control of our thoughts. Society burdens us with labels and imposes such ideas upon us, forcing us to direct our thoughts in the direction they are familiar with. This is what disables you from escaping this vicious cycle of society-imposed thoughts.

But there's a silver lining. There is a way out if only you are brave enough to understand and patient enough to embrace it.

It takes a great deal of courage to think differently from society, but the level of satisfaction that it brings along the peace that accompanies it is priceless.

For as long as I can remember, I have sown seeds of negative thoughts within myself. The negative emotions for my mother and the resentment I felt for my father were all rooted within me. I found that the hard way. I realized that instead of sowing so much negativity within, you need to fill yourself with limitless love, acknowledgment, and admiration for yourself.

And it all starts with a leap of faith.

As much as medicines and therapy are important in dealing with life's struggles, it's incomplete without your faith in yourself. We think having faith is a simple process—you start today, and by the end of the day, you feel better. However, it takes a lot more patience than this. Faith might be simple in theory. However, it's a lot easier said than done. It takes practice and patience in significant amounts before you actually start believing in your powers. But one thing I can assure you of is that it works its magic one day. You might not realize it, but soon, you open your eyes to the wonderful life you are surrounded by.

It is with faith that you open your mind to the concepts of self-compassion, self-love, and self-acceptance. These are the key ingredients that help you create a life that is fulfilling and satisfying. I spent far too many years fostering negative emotions for people, not caring about how it is impacting me from within.

Being diagnosed with a disease as horrendous as bipolar disorder is no ordinary man's task. Living with its horrors for years has helped me understand it in a way where I have some control over it. It was like living on the edge of a cliff. A single move was I needed to fall apart entirely. For normal people, sadness is just an overwhelming emotion. They cry and get it over with. For me, it could be life or death. It would take me one moment to destroy everything that I had strived so hard to achieve. The worst part of my life was the constant, lingering feeling of not being understood—neither my post-traumatic disorder stemming from childhood sexual abuse nor my brain's working after being diagnosed with bipolar disorder. All the time that I spent being angry at the world for not understanding me, I failed to realize that the only person who needed to understand and validate my feelings was no one else but myself.

It was not easy being blamed by my mother and the church for being molested, for being gas-lighted, a common practice of blaming the victims. Being heartbroken and failing to find peace or calm in life—things were challenging. My journey is like the tip of the iceberg. No matter how much I pen it down, it wouldn't reveal the depths. Only I can know the amount of suffering, trauma, loss, and breaking it took me to get here today, pouring down my darkest fears on a piece of paper.

Today, I stand here, tall, against my adversities, acknowledging my efforts and loving myself unconditionally. It took me decades of trauma, hurt, and heartbreak to realize that the only tools that would take me beyond my hardships were self-acceptance, self-acknowledgment, and non-judgment. I had to become comfortable in my own existence to be able to look beyond what and how the world looked upon or labeled me. Things did get easy for me, even when I thought it wouldn't.

You know what they say about diseases like diabetes and cancer; they have no cure. You can combat them with precautionary measures and management strategies. They require you to make some lifestyle changes in order to get better. The same thing applies to those who struggle with mental illnesses. The only thing with mental illnesses is that their scars are invisible. Nobody can feel them as strongly as you do. No one can be there for you as much as you can. Every word you utter becomes your heaven or grave. Your words act as a manifestation of your reality—a reality that you are capable of shaping.

It's often said that time is the largest single healer of mental scars. I'd be lying to myself if I said that was untrue. However, it isn't the only thing. Imagine a full garbage bag. What would happen if you kept filling it out? Eventually, its capacity to take trash would be filled, and it would no longer do its job. The trash would be lying all over the place, making the surroundings unhygienic. If one doesn't stop filling it soon, it would make everyone around it sick and nauseous. The same principle applies to our emotions. If we let the trash build up, thinking time will heal us, the garbage will keep increasing. There will come a time when your brain reaches its capacity. The trash will come outside, making the people around you unhappy.

The only trick here is to start emptying the trash at whatever chance you get. If you don't start, no one will come to your rescue. Because as much as you're reluctant to admit it, there's no saving from external forces. It's your job.

A famous quote from the legendary movie Spiderman says, "With great power comes great responsibility." You might think about what power has to do with mental struggles. Well, it has a lot to do with it. Your illnesses are the powers you haven't explored yet. I can only say this now: I am at a stage where I have made peace with my challenges. If you wish, you can certainly turn this disease into your superpower.

Often, we dive deep into the waters of self-judgment, critically analyzing and evaluating each step we take. I am not saying it's necessarily a bad thing. People should be able to keep themselves on a pedestal to ensure their progress. Nevertheless, when it comes to people who face mental health challenges, things might be a bit different. In the middle of criticizing, we forget that we are free-spirited beings. We don't have to measure and doubt every decision we make. We don't have to let our worst anticipation of the future hold us back from prospective goodness. Most importantly, we don't have to hop on the bandwagon of trending perspectives just for the sake of it. We need to embrace our uniqueness, be happy in our own skin, build our thought processes, and let life run its course. And for this, you need to perfect the art of self-compassion, self-love, and self-acceptance. Practicing compassion for yourself is necessary. Letting yourself be is a crucial step in the right direction. But the most important thing is to embrace the fact that you're worthy of every bit of love that the world has to offer.

Our pain cannot be measured on any scale. There's no way for me to express the intensity of the pain I felt. It cannot even be compared to the physical pain we feel. But now that I went through it, I feel the pain was important for me to experience. Otherwise, I wouldn't have looked at this life on a deeper level. I'd be searching for hollow notions and shallow lakes. To be frank with you, I like myself better this way. I wouldn't be so perceptive and intuitively aligned with my best interests if it weren't for the massive struggles I faced in my life. The bottom line here is to start accepting the situation for what it is. It's not an easy task by any means.

Honestly? It gets worse before it starts to get better. This is what my therapist would tell me all the time. I'd say, how much worse can it get than it already is? She would go silent. At that moment, her silence would aggravate the core of my existence, but now I know the reason she remained silent is because my question had no definitive answer. I got the answer through days and nights of contemplation—facing my worst instincts, letting my mind get the worst out of me.

We live in a world that has progressed in many ways, but in some cultures, mental health remains a stigma. The shame and guilt that the patients are put through can be brutal. It can shatter one's identity forever. However, let's go back to what I said in the beginning – nobody's coming to save you. Yes, people who love you might be there by your side to support you through your struggles, but saving yourself is your personal responsibility that no one else is capable of handling.

One thing that plays a magical role in your healing journey is self-awareness. The more you dig into the little parts of yourself, no matter how scary, the more you can help yourself. We might not be willing to show ourselves the mirror of reality when everything's falling apart. This is because of the fear of truth. Out of everyone, I should know how scary reality is, but that doesn't mean we stop trying. In order to get rid of the demons resting inside, we need to confront the truth about ourselves. We need to meet every little part in order to change the unwanted ones. The past patterns, the endless self-loathing, the betrayal—every wrong that we have committed needs to be unveiled to get closer to the beauty lying inside.

Additionally, making yourself aware of your illness also means being kind to yourself. Knowing that my disease did not define me as a person was an important part of my journey. It took me a significant time to learn that BPD was just a disease that I unfortunately crossed. It wasn't something that I chose.

It wasn't something I deliberately opted for. If anything, it was my genes and environment that worked alongside each other for me to inherit it.

I had to forgive myself for a crime I didn't commit.

Before this disease left my system, I had to release myself from the shackles of its bitterness.

I had to regain control of my life.

I had to stop from doing any more damage to myself.

At one point, it seemed meaningless for me to fight with this disease. It was as if I was fighting with an altar version of me. That's right. It was, in fact, an altar version—someone I had to learn to live with. Keeping the grip of hope tight, I let the vulnerability flow. I didn't escape it. Neither did I resist it. Instead, I let it hurt me until it couldn't. I let myself bleed until the dagger couldn't stab me. It was a long process and indeed a difficult one—to be this vulnerable. But it taught me my resilience. It made me realize the strength I am capable of. Remember when I mentioned the Spiderman quote? I found that my growth rested in vulnerability.

The roadblocks I experienced, in fact, laid the steps to a beautiful life.

III

The Complex Waters of Mental Health

"We live in a world that screams of human rights—respect, love, admiration, acceptance, yet get hushed when we show an ounce of concern over the stigma surrounding mental health. What a funny world it is."

\-   Amber Rae Johnson Diaz

Indeed, the irony of our society is laughable to its core. Is it a society that readily embraces change and accepts differences? No. Rather, it is a society that readily 'portrays' that it 'accepts' and 'embraces.' It is all for the show. It is people like us, trapped in the deep, dark dungeons of mental health problems, who know what a challenge it is to make people around us, even our loved ones, of what we are going through.

It is true when it is said, "Only the wearer knows where the shoe pinches."

No one will understand what an individual, sinking in the water of mental health instability, goes through every moment of their life.

How, in every living moment, all they can think about is ways to end their suffering?

How, at the end of their day, do they relive the moments they were judged for being the way they were?

How waking up and getting out of bed feels like climbing a mountain.

This comes from my experiences, my life's story—lined with episodes of bipolar disorder, post-traumatic disorder, anxiety, and restlessness.

Before you dive into the depths of mental health, it is important to understand what it actually is.

"Mental health is a state of mental well-being that enables people to cope with the stresses of life, realize their abilities, learn well and work well, and contribute to their community. It has intrinsic and instrumental value and is integral to our well-being."[1]

Instability of mental health translates to when an individual is unable to perform at their best due to failure to deal with the stresses of life. It makes it near to impossible to feel emotions such as joy, peace, calm, excitement, and even love. It gets in the way of every relationship one holds dear—leaving them alone, isolated, misunderstood, unheard, and, in worst cases, unloved and unwanted.

But is it just me and a few others?

Let's take a deeper dive into the statistics to reiterate the severity and seriousness of the mental health situation in not just our country but the entire world.

970 million people around the world struggle with some mental illness/drug abuse.[2]

14.3% of deaths worldwide, or approximately 8 million deaths each year, are attributable to mental disorders.[3]

---

[1] https://www.who.int/health-topics/mental-health#tab=tab_1
[2] https://www.who.int/health-topics/mental-health#tab=tab_2
[3] https://pubmed.ncbi.nlm.nih.gov/25671328/

Depression affects over 300 million people worldwide.[4]

This all may seem theoretical. Easier said than done, right?

Suicide is the third leading cause of death among people aged 15-29.[5]

284 million people suffer from an anxiety disorder worldwide.[6]

Now, let's get a bit close to home.

The United States has the highest global death rate from mental health issues.[7]

19.86% of adults are experiencing a mental illness, and 4.91% are experiencing a severe mental illness.[8]

Among U.S. adolescents aged 13-18, an estimated 49.5% of adolescents had any mental disorder.[9]

When the world is filled with millions of mental health patients, bombarded with victim stories of unstable mental health, why do people choose to stay quiet about it? Why is there a need to establish the mental health discussion as a taboo?

Do people like us not deserve to see the light at the end of the tunnel—the light that we hear every public speaker utter on international platforms, the light

---

[4] https://www.ncbi.nlm.nih.gov/pmc/articles/PMC9925363/#:~:text=Background,4%25%20of%20the%20world's%20population.

[5] https://www.who.int/news-room/fact-sheets/detail/suicide

[6] https://www.ncbi.nlm.nih.gov/pmc/articles/PMC10241552/

[7] https://www.commonwealthfund.org/publications/issue-briefs/2020/may/mental-health-conditions-substance-use-comparing-us-other-countries#:~:text=The%20United%20States%20has%20some,workers%2C%20particularly%20psychologists%20and%20psychiatrists.

[8] https://mhanational.org/issues/2022/mental-health-america-adult-data

[9] https://www.nimh.nih.gov/health/statistics/mental-illness

that literally is the basis of every motivational book ever written? Does this light only appear for those who have stable mental conditions?

Is there no end to our suffering?

Most of the mental disorders do not have a treatment.

- Bipolar disorder.
- Depression.
- Anxiety.
- Schizophrenia.
- Eating Disorders
- Obsessive-compulsive disorder (OCD).
- Post-traumatic stress disorder (PTSD).
- Impulse control disorder.
- Body dysmorphic disorder.
- Personality disorders.
- Dissociative disorder.

And the list goes on.

Why is it that our problems are not significant enough to garner the attention of the masses?

It is sad, disappointing, and downright unfair.

Anyone who is in the same boat as me—the boat carrying PTSD, bipolar disorder, depression, and anxiety—realizes how strong those who are able to live a beautiful life despite it.

I, for one, who was surrounded by such negative emotions due to my mental health problems, came out way stronger than I thought I could be. Though it was not my effort alone that helped me, I had accountability partners, unconventional healing methodologies, and, of course, medicines and therapy; it was my will to stand tall. It was my resilient personality that pushed me to fight—fight not just the demons outside but also those within me. It was scary and was not easy.

I lost interest in things I once loved to do.

I had a rough and close to terrible relationship with my parents.

I lived through the worst of heartbreaks.

But did it stop me from building my life? Even though I realized my true power was embedded in my resilience, vulnerability, and self-acceptance a bit late, I welcomed the ideas wholeheartedly. I am not going to sugarcoat things for you; there are a lot of external factors that play their part, but it is YOU who decide. It is YOU who welcomes the idea. It is YOU who opens themselves to the possibility of healing. Sticking to those tired, old strategies is not how you can rebuild your life. You need to be open to unconventional approaches. Reiterating what I said earlier, there is no such thing as one-size-fits-all when it comes to healing. You need to look around, acknowledge your emotions, study your feelings, and check for your triggers—this is what leads you to discover of your way to heal.

Spending most of my life looking for validation from others around me, relying on my supposed loved ones to catch me when I fell, and blaming others for my situation brought nothing but disappointment, shattered expectations, and a void within that I just could not fill. The void that was created due to my mental health disorders and issues was not something I was born with. It was a void that was created after living a major part of my life dealing with unimaginable issues.

My childhood? It was anything but ideal. My mother, as talked about earlier, did not care much about what was going on in my life. Sexual abuse? Being molested by my stepfather? It was all my fault. Dealing with a father who was least interested in my life, enjoying his time with his other family. Being a rock for my siblings—not a childhood one would not dream of.

So, adverse childhood experiences, **check.**

Trauma and stressful situations, **check.**

Being ignored by loved ones, the feeling of isolation, **check.**

Severe, long-term stress, **check.**

These were just a few of the triggers that exposed me to the risks of mental health disorders. I was not ready to deal with it, which is why I found the way to recovery later in life. If you're worried about your mental health disorders, you are not the one to be blamed. What is to be blamed are the factors that led you to it and the factors that triggered it. Childhood trauma, societal neglect, too many responsibilities, genetic roots—anything can lead you to the deep dungeon of mental health disorders.

Unfortunately, diagnoses of mental health illnesses or disorders are not that straightforward. Blood tests can be used to identify heart diseases, and measuring blood glucose levels helps with the diagnosis of diabetes. X-rays can help identify fractures, while ultrasounds can capture imagery of internal injuries. But there are no blood tests, X-rays, or medical tests that can help identify mental health disorders. This brings me to the point where I tell you that the first step of diagnosis is to be done on your own. As mental health issues are so common all across the globe, analyzing your mental state for disorders or illnesses is not an overreaction. However, being paranoid is not the right way to go about it.

Some of the most common early signs of mental health conditions are hidden in some day-to-day feelings—the only difference is the persistence of these feelings.

- Distancing yourself from your loved ones, family, and friends
- Not finding joy in activities you once enjoyed
- Disturbed circadian cycle/sleeping cycle: too much to too little sleep
- Problems in eating: too much or too less
- Lingering feelings of hopelessness
- Functioning with a constant low energy level
- Outburst of negative feelings or emotions
- Finding yourself confused more often
- Reduced motivation or energy to complete daily tasks
- Urge to self-harm

If you find yourself experiencing most of these or all, the next step is to head to a mental health professional. You cannot self-diagnose. When I got diagnosed with bipolar disorder, it made me feel like it was the end of the world. The feeling that the people I love could not trust me with emotions, suddenly becoming the most unreliable and unpredictable person in the room, pushed me to an all-time low. This is where my accountability partners, such as my therapist, the people at the church, my friends, and different healing methodologies, came into the picture. All of these elements, along with my willpower to survive through this—embrace my situation, acknowledge my condition, and build a life alongside it—allowed me to be where I am today.

Just know that *you are not alone,* and your will and desire to move past it and be open to different ways of healing will take you a long way!

IV

There's No One-Size-Fits-All

"Healing is a very personal journey—it takes no influences, it is not shared between two individuals, it is a unique path for every person."

-          Amber Rae Johnson Diaz

If I say that life cannot be more beautiful than it is when you are healed, it won't be an exaggeration. I am not, in any way, sugarcoating the reality. What good would it do to me, right? This is something I have experienced myself, and I would not trade it for anything else in this world. For me, there is no going back—not in a negative way, but a desire to witness life's beauty at its best now that I am on my healing journey.

Honestly? I just cannot stop, and I won't stop until I have fully healed.

My healing journey has opened a doorway to a kind of life that revolved around true joy, peace of mind, and calmness of the soul. Just a glimpse, and I am in awe.

Could life be this beautiful? One can only wonder.

So many of us find ourselves struggling to survive, struggling to make it to the next day—for us, life is a burden, a punishment that we need to complete. A sentence to decades of agony. How can we come to believe that there's a way to experience true joy in this world? Sounds impossible.

It was the same for me.

Not in my wildest thoughts did I think that my life could be better, could be joyful, and even satisfying. After all, there was nothing I had to make me think otherwise. A broken family. A mother too obsessed with her work. A father who did not care. A world that was nothing but unkind to me.

But today, I sit here, penning down my experiences, on my way to becoming an author—did I even think I could do this? Here I am, living a life even better than my dreams. I am excited to start my nursing training center; I am thrilled to build my resort with a gym, private jet, Jacuzzi, and everything people like me would need to relax and unwind. I have big dreams; I wish to make it big in life.

From being suicidal to brewing such big dreams, I have come a long way. And how did I do it? I curated my own path toward healing.

I identified my weaknesses.

I analyzed my vulnerabilities.

I spotted my triggers.

I built up my will to come out stronger from my adversities—**I chose to heal.**

It is important to understand that you cannot expect nature and the usual course of life to heal you. Healing is a choice. You take charge of your life, stand tall on your feet, and you push yourself to find a way out. It won't just happen. You cannot just sit and wait for the universe to start working in your favor—it will never happen.

You have to choose to heal.

Acknowledging that you need to heal to live life better is the first step in the right direction; the second is understanding that this journey is personal and has to be walked alone. Walking alone means that no one will share this journey with you. There will be your loved ones around, but how you heal is something they would not understand. Be it your closely-knit family, best friend, or even your spouse. Every person is unique in their nature, which requires completely different approaches toward living life and doing things. One of the most critical factors in the process of healing is understanding that there's no one-size-fits-all approach toward healing.

It is pretty common to hear from your loved ones about how they overcame a challenge in their lives or came out of a situation stronger. While they do this out of love and merely to help us in our difficult times, it usually is of no help. For instance, if a person was diagnosed with depression and insomnia and it was the right medication that helped them get better, it does not necessarily mean that others would enjoy the same results. There are chances that medication may produce side effects in their life that may hinder their growth, making things worse for them.

Every person in this world is part of a unique storyline with completely different approaches to living life. So, the third step of the process is to stop comparing your way and pace of healing with those around you. Each person has a different path toward finding that light at the end of the tunnel, and you need to find yours.

Some people come across the best ways to deal with the challenges in life and find their way out in the earliest possible timeframe, while others spend decades in the search. I found my path toward healing very later in life. It did not happen overnight; I did not just wake up one day knowing that this was how I would heal. As I moved forward in life, things started opening up for me. While I am not the most successful person in the world or someone you need to follow in order to make it big in life, embrace peace, calm, and joy. I am merely one of the millions of examples out there. The only difference is that I have chosen to share it with you.

Many of you might find comfort in doing things that others may frown upon or not prefer doing. The same is the case with healing. Despite what people around you say, if going about a certain way is allowing you to find inner satisfaction and peace, that is your way to get better, your pathway towards a healed version of yourself. You need to be strong and courageous enough to accept it.

Tori Amos, an American music artist, once said, *"Healing takes courage, and we all have courage, even if we have to dig a little to find it."*

The reason why I have decided to share my journey toward healing is to spread the word that one has to be courageous and patient enough to welcome new ideas into one's life. They need to be open to their emotions—they need to be transparent about how they feel. Letting society or your loved ones decide how you go about living life to achieve that inner satisfaction and joy is one of the biggest mistakes you can make.

I can break down my healing journey into five elements: submission and surrender, spiritual growth, self-care, accountability partners, and medicines.

While most people agree that diving into one's spirituality, prioritizing yourself, surrounding yourself with people who love you, and medicines can help one get better, not many understand that submission and surrendering are healing tools. Again, I do not wish anyone to 'understand' how I heal, but it is important to share it with the world and to open their minds to endless possibilities when it comes to healing.

I found a sense of calm in surrendering and submission when I was introduced to the concepts of BDSM: Bondage, Discipline (or Dominance), Submission (or Sadism), and Masochism. Yes, it is something society frowns upon; it is considered a negative practice in various places across the world, but it came to me as a way to comfort. My dating life is no less than a bumpy ride, but it offered me the exposure to explore the idea of BDSM. There were two dominants in my life: Shira, a sensual dominant, and Shana, a sadist dominant. Both of them opened an entirely different room for me. Did I even think about BDSM as a way to heal? As a way to move on from my past traumas? Never in my life did I think that my vulnerability would make my life better in unimaginable ways. As mentioned earlier, I was sexually violated when I was just a child—it made me feel powerless and weak. I was molested by a man as old as my father—my stepfather. What could a little girl like me do in a situation like this? This is where BDSM comes into the picture.

BDSM helps address this traumatic experience of life. It is no wonder that my PTSD stems from this horrendous part of my life. Being sexually abused and molested in childhood really messed up my mind. But it was after being introduced to the idea of consensual submission and surrendering that I regained control. The way my childhood experiences made me feel powerless, this practice allows me to set my own terms of submission—where my partner knows exactly what I want and don't want.

I understand how hard it may be for people to wrap their heads around this, but the purpose of my sharing these details is to make you understand that healing is a unique experience for every individual. The key here is to be open to all ideas and carefully break down the feelings and emotions of different activities in your life to be able to understand how doing one thing impacts your mind.

If I had not been honest with myself and would have cared about what society would think of me, I would not be here, writing my story and helping you and countless others to find their way to healing. I was courageous enough to acknowledge my feelings, and this is exactly what led me to my healing mechanism.

Would I change anything about it? **Never.**

V

Submission and Surrender: What's The Deal?

" Being vulnerable is not a weakness—even the most powerful humans have gone through some of their darkest phases. "

- Amber Rae Johnson Diaz

Vulnerability is often misunderstood as a weakness, but it's actually a strength that fosters trust, intimacy, and meaningful relationships. Think about the people you feel most comfortable with—those who make you feel loved and accepted. These connections thrive because they are rooted in trust and emotional honesty.

Take, for example, the song Alone by Alan Walker. Its heartfelt lyrics resonate with millions because they speak to our shared vulnerability:

"Cause you are that someone

That gets me like no one else

Right when I need it the most

And I'll be the one you rely on

A shoulder to cry on

A friend through the highs and the lows."

This universal need for connection reminds us that being vulnerable isn't just okay—it's essential. Vulnerability extends beyond everyday relationships.

Whether in love, friendships, or intimate fantasies, vulnerability builds bridges, not walls. Embrace it—it's your strength.

I realized this later in life… much later.

I often wondered why I was so fragile while others seemed super strong. I never considered myself worthy enough to be loved. What else can you expect from a person who was neglected by their own parents? I was molested sexually by a person who was my father's age, and when I complained about it to my mother, guess what happened? The victim was blamed.

That day, the innocent Amber was lost in the chaos of this world.

After this specific incident, I found myself surrounded by vulnerabilities.

For a decade or more, I was quiet or, more appropriately, ignored. I kept reminding myself that you must justify the traditional definition of a "Strong Person."

"Who is strong, less to no emotional and non-vulnerable. He fights, and in most cases-dominates too."

I tried and failed, again and again, until I gave up.

I was lost in self-blame and disappointment, but that changed when I met—Shira, a sensual dominant, and Shana, a sadist. It was through them that I discovered BDSM for the first time.

Because they were dominant, I happily chose to surrender and submit. For the very first time in my life, I felt relaxed and understood. Someone was there who was okay with my flaws; most importantly, it happened with my consent.

I was informed – understood – loved and cared for.

There was no one to blame me for my dark thoughts of surrender.

There are multiple facets of life where vulnerability and trust play a central role, BDSM (Bondage and Discipline, Dominance and Submission, Sadism and Masochism) being one of them. Through open communication and consent, partners explore submission and surrender, discovering a deeper connection. For instance, a submissive consent to surrender control, while the dominant ensures their safety and comfort. This dynamic, when approached responsibly, celebrates vulnerability as a pathway to trust and intimacy.

You may relate or may not, but let me walk you through my personal experiences of how surrendering and submitting helped me to heal. It was when I embraced my vulnerability that I was able to see beyond and find a kind of comfort and peace in surrendering and submission.

Unfortunately, the society that we live in makes it impossible for one to enjoy the many hidden healing benefits of not-so-traditional methodologies, such as BDSM.

Society whispers: Don't cry; it's weakness.

It warns: Don't feel it'll hurt you.

It demands: Don't care; it makes you fragile.

Aren't we tired of "don't be too this or too that?" Yes, we are.

So, here I am, penning down my journey of healing through not-so-common-ways.

That, too, by being submissive throughout the journey. I have never transitioned from submissive to dominant. I am comfortable with who I am and what I want.

It was with my experiences that I discovered that I love to surrender and feel the fantasies of submission. By putting my trust in someone in the most intimate situation, I was able to find the ray of light that guided me to the point where I am today.

As you know, I had always struggled with trust, burdened by past trauma that left me feeling fragile and afraid to open up. Then I met Shira, who gently introduced me to the idea of BDSM—not as something harsh, but as a way to heal.

We started small, with a soft scarf loosely wrapped around my wrists. It wasn't about restraint; it was about letting go in a safe space, knowing I could stop whenever needed. Slowly, I learned that bondage was about release, not control.

Next, she showed me the comfort of discipline—not as punishment, but to create structure. We set playful rules, which made me feel seen and understood, free from judgment.

When we explored submission, I found unexpected relief in letting someone else guide me—within the limits I set. It wasn't about giving up power but about trusting myself to communicate my boundaries.

That's how I faced my fears through the safe exploration of sadism and masochism. It wasn't about pain but about reclaiming my voice—learning to say "stop" or "go" without fear. I felt alive, respected, and, indeed, in control in those moments.

I not only discovered but experienced that BDSM wasn't about losing myself—it was about choosing how, when, and who to trust. It was about reclaiming my power, one safe step at a time.

After every session, my perception of the world began to change. I liked the direction I was going in; it was brewing hope within me.

I have come to this conclusion after multiple attempts: I was a GOOD GIRL first, who followed everything that came her way.

They suggested sharing—I asked with whom—with my mother, who doesn't care, or my father, whose existence is as good as non-existing?

After going through multiple paths and walking past a million steps, I always concluded that this wasn't helping. It was as simple as that.

Wandering was always destined for me—and so was finding the destination.

And my path toward my healed self was BDSM; for many, it's a dark place, even a taboo. However, for me, it's the safest and most effective healing practice I have discovered with my two dominants.

It may sound dark to you, but BDSM is based upon the principles of YOGA, breathwork, rhythm, and repetition. A large body of evidence shows how valuable breath work can be in helping depression and anxiety and regulating the nervous system.[10]

Similarly, rhythm and repetition of the same actions helped me build trust and a sense of security.

---

[10] https://www.cbc.ca/life/wellness/from-fight-or-flight-to-rest-and-digest-how-to-reset-your-nervous-system-with-the-breath-1.4485695#:~:text=Breathing%20deeply%2C%20with%20a%20slow,heartbeat%20and%20shallow%20chest%20breathing.

I was molested and humiliated not once but twice. I always wanted to speak loudly about them in an echo chamber, and I never found one (Until BDSM). I was suffocating inside; I had a lot of oxygen to breathe in but not enough capacity to keep doing it.

At first, I was hesitant, like many of you, as we have misunderstood it with painful sex or, in the worst cases, with pedophilia. You may be shocked after knowing that BDSM is not only about sex; people with high involvement reported that 35% of the time, it is non-sexual fun-play for them to release tension from their day-to-day life.

It's more like a power play between submissive and dominant; that's why we have multiple plays, including bondage, humiliation, sensation play, impact play, role play, acts of service, and more. It is not and cannot be an inhuman activity. Since consent was included in the written form,

Before practicing BDSM with Shira, we both were in the talking stage—trying our best to understand each other. Even our second stage was impractical; we signed a contract stating what we both wanted and how we wanted after agreeing to everything we did in our first session.

It was all about sensory pleasures, relaxation, and submitting myself to someone whom I could trust.

The purpose of my tapping into such a personal journey is not for the world to know what I did but to instill hope in the hearts of those who have given up on their healing journey. Of course, healing is not an overnight process—but a gradual one. The results are often slow, but with time, things begin to fall into place. While many people find ways to heal in the traditional ways, I want to share with the world that they have to be open to all and every kind of possibility.

Just like I found comfort and mental peace in embracing my vulnerable self and accepting the fact that my submissive behavior and surrendering power will lead my way further in my healing journey, you can find yours!

You just have to keep an open mind.

VI

You Can Never Overlook Spirituality

"The genuine world extends beyond the realms of wealth, fame, and power—the domain where spirituality resides."

-                    Amber Rae Johnson Diaz

As I reflect on my healing journey, numerous factors have keyed in and enabled me to grow more comfortable in my own skin. Spirituality is one of the paramount reasons I was able to reconcile with myself and confront my darkest sides as I took a seat to pen down my story for the world to read.

The interpretation of spirituality varies from person to person; for some, it's rooted in religious observance; for others, it's about connecting with nature, practicing yoga, engaging in fitness, participating in community service, and so forth.

For me, however, spirituality fundamentally means striking a harmonious balance between religious and secular practices. Yes, I committed myself to church at the tender age of ten and even began meditation at a very young age.

I explored and immersed myself in every conceivable method to heal. My relationship with God allowed me to rely on a being far greater than myself. God, Who consistently formulates better plans for me.

I experienced a profound sense of contentment and a remarkable surge in my self-esteem whenever I laid bare my tear-streaked heart before Him.

Was I always this way? No.

Did I consciously work towards becoming this person? Absolutely.

We have all endured phases in our lives when we were vulnerable, aimless…, and too fragile to envision doing something constructive for ourselves. We despise ourselves for who we are, where we come from, and, most importantly, why we exist.

I have now found comprehensive answers to these questions—albeit belatedly—but I have them.

Have you ever sat with yourself in the dead of the night when the world is asleep, and only you and your inner self remain, burdened with guilt, traumas, and suffering? Moments so excruciating that it's hard to even draw breath.

I have, and as I write this, tears of joy blur my vision.

The term 'spirituality' transports me to the time I first encountered the essence of true love, when I first sensed the presence of God, when I first cradled my daughter, when I committed to a gym membership, when I enrolled in the nursing academy when I dreamt of writing this book, and when I named myself as a *Black Diamond*—rare and invaluable.

One morning, not long ago, I was leaving my home for work when I noticed a teenager taking a morning stroll—without a phone, earphones, or a sugary drink. Pretty common for the generation of today. And I was taken aback.

Do you know what it reminded me of? **Spirituality**.

We, as humans, are multifaceted—a complex fusion of distinct experiences and choices, aren't we? We can't impose a uniform spiritual experience on everyone. For me, spirituality is distinct; for you, it might be different, and that's perfectly acceptable.

That teenager was embodying what we now call 'Modern Spirituality,' or 'Environmentalism,' a movement that fosters a profound connection to our planet and nature. Contemporary spirituality is more approachable and, in many ways, slightly more effective than traditional forms.

How can we expect a mother, overwhelmed with the demands of toddlers, to dedicate two hours to a yoga session? Does that mean she doesn't deserve to be at the pinnacle of mental well-being? It would be rude to dictate a single pathway to healing. For her, the ideal scenario might be to join an online community of like-minded individuals and access everything she needs at her fingertips.

At this juncture, I'd like to share a well-known quote by Emma Watson.

"I'm interested in spirituality and deeply interested in what it means to be a human being. I'm not interested in anything other than truth."

We all recognize Emma from the celebrated Harry Potter series as Hermione Granger, but is that all she is known for? Emma is among the few individuals who unearthed their authentic selves at a remarkably young age. Today, she is not merely a successful actress but a person who has earned a place in our hearts. She embraced spirituality through her volunteer work for humanitarian causes. She cherishes humanity for its own sake. In her narrative, spirituality is about alleviating pain for others, even if all you have to offer are words.

Just do it!

It takes me back to the day I surrendered myself to Jesus at ten years old. I was anxious and apprehensive, bearing burdens that were heavy to carry but not easy to relinquish. The moment I submitted to a higher power, all I felt was profound relief and solace.

Someone who possesses knowledge of the past, present, and future simultaneously; who orchestrated my existence and the universe; who predestined my fate long before I was born; who loves me beyond any conceivable measure.

How could it be possible that He would 'err-ed' in my life's course?

How beautiful it is to have blind trust in God.

The greatest gift we receive from having an ally like God is serenity—the assurance in our life choices, the decisions we make, and the paths we choose to follow. That faith emboldens us before the entire human race and enables us to adhere to our convictions resolutely.

It renders our vulnerable moments and darkest periods more tolerable. It strengthens us with the mindset that 'This Too Shall Pass.' After all, every hardship comes with relief, and after every pitch-black night, a dazzling dawn awaits.

Healing is a journey—often a lengthy one—if you cannot run, then walk; if you cannot walk, then crawl; but maintain your momentum—slow or fast, does it really matter?

Believe it or not, cultivating genuine faith in God or a higher power isn't a challenging task; all it requires is the surrender of your ego—the abandonment of your darker side—the relinquishment of everything impeding your healing process.

Once you surrender and begin to accept, "I can be wrong—I can be imperfect—I can be vulnerable—I can be broken," all the fragments of the puzzle will eventually align, leading you to your ultimate calling, which declares, "There's a long road ahead to become the individual I aspire to be."

"I have held many things in my hands, and I have lost them all, whatever I have placed in God's hands, that I still possess."

— Martin Luther.

Spirituality is a deeply personal journey, and no two paths are the same. At this very point, I want to provide you with some exercises in spiritual reflection, prayer, and contemplation to help you connect with what resonates most with you.

Whether you are drawn to traditional religious practices, the beauty of nature, or your own personal exploration, these exercises are designed to guide you in finding what brings you peace and fulfillment.

Take these exercises at your own pace, and remember that spirituality is as unique as you are. Keep exploring, be patient with yourself, and let your path unfold naturally.

Start Practicing Mindfulness Meditation:

I understand you guys are not experts and cannot start with something tricky. So, meditation is a great start for many of you to heal from traumas you have been carrying for years. Find a quiet space, sit comfortably, and close your eyes. Focus on your breath as you inhale and exhale slowly. If your mind wanders, gently bring it back to your breath.

Exercise: Dedicate 5-10 minutes each day to mindfulness meditation. Begin by noticing your breathing. Pay attention to how each breath feels, where your mind goes, and how your body responds.

Don't worry! If it doesn't align with you, simply choose another one.

Remember, every person has a unique way to heal.

Embracing Nature as a Spiritual Practice:

Nature has a unique way of connecting us to something beyond ourselves. It can be a grounding force, a reminder of the cycles of life, and a source of beauty and wonder. Spend time in nature—walk in the woods, sit by a river, or visit a local park. Let the sights, sounds, and smells draw you out of your mind and into the present moment.

<u>Exercise:</u> Go for a walk and pick a small object that catches your eye—a leaf, a stone, or a flower. Sit with this object and observe it closely. What colors, textures, and patterns do you notice? Reflect on how this small piece of nature fits into the larger world and what it means to you.

Creating Space for Prayer:

For those who resonate with traditional religion, like my former self, prayer can be a powerful way to connect spiritually.

<u>Exercise:</u> Set aside a few minutes each day to pray. Use this time to focus on gratitude, seek guidance, or simply express your thoughts to a higher power or the universe. If you're unsure how to start, consider:

Until this point, I have listed traditional factors only. I highly encourage you to try many of them and stick with one which you find most effective. If all the traditional methods fail to give you what you want, then you can opt for something non-traditional, just like myself. Trust me, the right way to heal will find you if you stay consistent in your efforts.

It is a trial-and-error method and works only if you're truly determined to make things better for yourself.

As I navigated my path toward healing, I found BDSM. Contrary to popular belief, it served as a powerful tool for healing and personal growth for me. It helped me explore aspects of my untouched self, confront trauma, and build trust in a way that is both safe and consensual.

Healing through spirituality is an intensely personal journey. I cannot foresee what might resonate with you, just as you cannot predict what will be effective for me. To gain a deeper understanding of your own mind, begin by engaging in the exercises I outlined earlier. They are straightforward to grasp and uncomplicated enough to maintain consistency. Remember, you are valuable, and you deserve to experience the best version of yourself, just as I did.

The timing—whether sooner or later—is irrelevant; what matters is that you proceed at your own pace. Embrace spirituality as fully as you can.

VII

Don't Forget to Tap Into the Power of Self-Care

" If They Call You Selfish, Prove Them Right."

- Amber Rae Johnson Diaz

Self-care. You've heard it before. It's all over social media, in wellness newsletters, and in conversations about "living your best life." But let's be honest—how many of us actually do it, actually take care of ourselves? Do you not just talk about it or post a #SelfCareSunday selfie but truly practice it, day in and day out?

For most of us, the answer is not enough.

And why? Because we overcomplicate it. We think it's about lavish spa treatments, expensive gym memberships, or hours of meditation. But what if I told you that true self-care doesn't require any of that? It can start right where you are, with what you already have.

So, let's redefine self-care with me. Self-care isn't about luxury; it's about necessity. It's the small, intentional acts that nurture your body, mind, and soul.

Imagine this:

- Taking a 10-minute walk in the morning sun.

- Savoring a quiet cup of tea before the day's chaos begins.
- Write down your thoughts in a journal instead of letting them spiral in your head.

Self-care is all about small actions with big impacts.

So, why do we ignore self-care?

If you're like most people, self-care probably feels like an afterthought. We tend to prioritize it only after something goes wrong—after losing a loved one, experiencing a breakup, or facing a health scare. I've been there, too. I didn't start taking self-care seriously until my late twenties. And while it might feel "late," I've learned that it's always better to start now than never.

I'm not here to preach perfection. I'm here because I believe in the power of transformation. My goal isn't to sell you quick fixes. It's to inspire lasting change. If even one person reading this book decides to prioritize their well-being, it will have been worth it.

Impact over income. That's my guiding principle.

I understand human psychology well—we often thrive under pressure, relying on do-or-die situations to push us toward major achievements. But here's the truth: self-care isn't a luxury; it's a necessity. Let me walk you through fact-based, well-researched reasons that prove why taking care of yourself is not just important but essential.

Let's talk about what happens when we don't prioritize self-care.

Premature Death: The World Health Organization (WHO) estimates that regular physical activity could prevent 3.9 million early deaths each year.

Imagine how many dreams, goals, and connections are lost because people don't prioritize their health.[11]

Stress: A survey by YouGov revealed that nearly half of respondents felt less stressed when they engaged in self-care. A calm mind often leads to better decisions, healthier relationships, and a happier life.[12]

Burnout: Work-life balance isn't a luxury; it's essential. When we fail to balance our responsibilities, burnout becomes inevitable.

Relationships: Taking care of yourself makes you better for others. When you're emotionally balanced, you can communicate clearly, set boundaries, and nurture deeper connections.

Self-Esteem: How often do you feel unworthy because you've neglected yourself? Self-care helps shift that narrative. It reminds you that you are deserving of love, respect, and joy.

And here's the thing: neglecting yourself doesn't just affect you. It affects your relationships, your work, and your ability to fully participate in life.

To truly embrace self-care, we first need to release ourselves from the invisible chains of societal expectations. The belief that you don't deserve love? It's a lie that thrives on these imposed standards. The truth is simple: you are deserving of love, rest, and grace—no conditions attached.

It's okay to feel unproductive. It's okay to feel anxious.

Life is not a linear path, and neither is healing. What's not okay, however, is to let these feelings take root and grow unchecked.

---

[11]   https://www.thelancet.com/journals/langlo/article/PIIS2214-109X(20)30211-4/fulltext

[12]   https://business.yougov.com/content/50132-32-of-us-adults-engage-in-daily-self-care-practices

So, how long is too long? That depends on you. If you once needed three days to bounce back from a setback but now only need one, celebrate that progress. You've evolved.

Now that we understand why self-care matters, let's discuss how to make it part of your life—not as a fleeting commitment but as a lasting habit.

I've broken it down into three stages: Alpha, Beta, and Gamma. Think of them as levels in a game. Each one builds on the last, helping you progress toward a life where self-care is second nature.

But before we dive in, let's set one thing straight: there's no rush. This isn't about speed. It's about progress.

Stage 1: The Alpha Stage

This is your starting point. It's where you build the foundation, focusing on the basics: physical and emotional well-being. These are the cornerstones of self-care. Without them, it's hard to move forward in any other area of life.

Your affirmations for this stage:

"I am worthy of care."

"I deserve to feel good."

<u>Physical Self-Care:</u>

- Prioritize rest. Sleep isn't a luxury—it's essential.
- Nourish your body with wholesome foods.
- Move. A 20-minute walk, some stretching, or a dance session in your living room—anything that gets you moving.

<u>Emotional Self-Care:</u>

- Journal. Start with a few sentences each day. Write what you feel, what you want, what you're grateful for.

- Express your emotions. Cry if you need to. Laugh freely. Hug someone you love.

- Read something that inspires you, even if it's just one page.

You can't pour from an empty cup. Taking care of your body and emotions gives you the energy and clarity to handle life's challenges.

Once you've started nurturing your body and emotions, something interesting happens: You begin to feel a sense of stability. That's your cue to move to the next stage—the Beta Stage. But before we go there, take a moment to acknowledge your progress.

Small steps lead to big wins.

Stage 2: The Beta Stage

This stage is about expansion. Now that you've laid a solid foundation, it's time to nurture other aspects of your life: spiritual, social, and financial well-being.

These areas are interconnected. Think about it:

A strong spiritual foundation gives you inner strength—healthy social connections provide support and inspiration—and financial stability reduces stress and opens doors to opportunities.

Your affirmations for this stage:

"I am growing in all areas of my life."

"I have the strength to balance and thrive."

Spiritual Self-Care:

- Practice gratitude. Focus on what you have, not what you lack.

- Find moments of stillness. Whether it's prayer, meditation, or simply sitting quietly, connect with something bigger than yourself.

<u>Social Self-Care:</u>

- Reconnect with old friends.
- Volunteer. Helping others often helps us feel more connected and fulfilled.
- Practice kindness in small ways—say "thank you" and smile often.

<u>Financial Self-Care:</u>

- Set a small savings goal. Even $10 a week adds up.
- Update your resume. Invest in your professional growth.
- Be mindful of spending. Focus on what truly brings value to your life.

When you nurture these areas, you create a life that feels balanced and meaningful.

You're building momentum now. As you strengthen your spiritual, social, and financial well-being, you'll notice a shift in your mindset. You'll feel more grounded and more capable. That's when you're ready for the final stage—the Gamma Stage.

Stage 3: The Gamma Stage

This stage is about mastery. It's where you refine and protect your most valuable assets: your mind and your career.

Your affirmations for this stage:

"I am in control of my growth."

"I invest in my future with intention."

<u>Intellectual Self-Care:</u>

- Consume content that challenges and inspires you—books, podcasts, courses.
- Explore creativity. What hobby have you always wanted to try? Now's the time.

<u>Occupational Self-Care:</u>

- Invest in professional development.
- Advocate for yourself—ask for that raise or promotion.
- Set clear goals and take actionable steps toward them.

Mastery of your mind and career opens doors to limitless possibilities. It's about living life on your terms.

If this feels overwhelming (though it really isn't), try tackling it with an "accountability partner." Trust me, having someone to check in with can make all the difference. Over the years, I've had several accountability partners, each playing a crucial role at different stages of my life. Their support has been invaluable. It's a simple but powerful addition to your productivity toolkit.

As you move through these stages, remember this: motivation is fleeting. Discipline is lasting. It's what keeps you going when the excitement fades, and life gets tough.

You've got everything you need to thrive. Start small. Stay consistent. Trust the process. Most importantly, you should know that you are worth every bit of care and effort you give yourself.

VIII

Does This Mean No Medicines?

"There's no shame in mental illness; the shame lies in a society that stigmatizes it."

- Amber Rae Johnson Diaz

When I first discovered I was battling with bipolar disorder, I was utterly shaken. For the longest time, I had mistaken my mental health struggles for mere 'mood swings' toward the extreme end of the scale. Never did it cross my mind that I could be one of those fighting with a mental health condition, that, too, bipolar disorder.

The thought haunted me: Am I so fragile that I was diagnosed with this disorder?

This very question inspired me to dedicate this chapter to my journey. Pause for a moment and reflect on my question. Notice how unconsciously I equate my vulnerability with weakness. This very narrative has deep roots in our society about mental illness.

Isn't this the same stigma our society clings to? We casually dismiss terms like "depression" and "anxiety," dividing the world into two camps: those who make fun of these struggles, labeling every minor setback as a cause for anxiety, and those genuinely suffering from profound mental disorders, too ashamed to seek help for fear of being branded as "weak."

Why this hesitance? Because society often labels people with mental illness as weak individuals and not normal. Whenever we as individuals get to know that our friend, colleague, or spouse is suffering from a mental disorder, we start trusting them less, and we start treating them differently. At the time when they needed us the most, we left them alone.

This was my reality.

At one of my prior jobs, I lived under the delusion that we were a family. But the moment they discovered my bipolar disorder, they severed ties completely, terminating my employment and abandoning our so-called "family bond." It left me questioning.

Was it ever real?

Would family leave you in your darkest hours?

True family, those who genuinely care for you, don't turn their backs when you struggle. Their love and support are unconditional.

So, why let the judgment of a society that abandons you in moments of vulnerability dictate your worth? Why give them the power to influence your decisions?

Are they worth it? No, they aren't.

And yet, there's another myth why people are afraid of consulting doctors, which is that mental illness is permanent and can't be cured. Now, you have to live with it. You'll often hear, "Once you have it, there's no cure." Most of these voices lack even a basic understanding of mental health, yet they feel entitled to preach.

Let me debunk this whole topic here. If your mind asks you why, Amber? I am the one who has experienced not one but multiple mental illnesses all at once. I am the one who has recovered from all this. My experiences are personal and effective. I am not a doctor, but I am a survivor.

So, my few words are that you cannot get rid of your mental illness completely. Still, you can reduce the symptoms to a minimum by choosing effective therapies, medications, and consultations.

Medication alone is not enough, of course. Cure for mental illness lies in the compound effect of medication + therapies + brain stimulation + self-care. This combo varies for every individual.

People often challenge me, saying, "Why should I invest money in something like mental health?" My response is simple: mental health is foundational. It impacts every facet of your life. Your career, relationships, and overall well-being. Ignore it now and prepare yourself for a difficult future. Overlooking your well-being is the worst mistake you can make in life.

I want you to know that there's a world as beautiful as your imagination, where:

- You excel at work without any mood swings.

- Your relationships flourish as your concentration improves.

- Your finances stabilize because you're more grounded in reality.

- Your days become more productive, free from exhaustion and sleeping problems.

This isn't a fairy tale. It's the reality awaiting you once you prioritize your mental health. You don't need to be "cured" completely to see transformative results.

The journey equips you with resilience and clarity to tackle challenges head-on.

The best thing we lose in the suffering of mental illness is our self-control. Our ability to think, brainstorm, and perform our best. So, our main target would be to regain self-control, and everything would follow it eventually.

But how do you know when it's time to seek help?

My answer is simple. Our body gives us signals. I can't trust if you're saying that you have developed this condition within a few months or weeks. It's not possible. Your body displayed signs for a long time; however, you chose to ignore it completely. There is a list of signals that sends you a message that it is enough now and it's time to consult with a doctor, which includes:

- Persistent sadness.

- Difficulty concentrating or making decisions.

- Constant feeling of guilt.

- Extreme mood swings.

- Withdrawal from social activities.

- Tiredness and sleeping problems.

- Detachment from reality and living in delusion.

- Difficulty coping with daily stresses.

- Change in sex drive.

- Suicidal thoughts.

Even one of these symptoms warrants consultation. Delaying action to save money now could lead to higher costs and suffering later.

Recovery requires a multi-disciplinary team:

- A pharmacist to manage medications.

- A family doctor to oversee your general health.

- Supportive family members to provide emotional stability.

- A psychiatrist to diagnose and treat your condition.

- A psychotherapist to guide you through therapy.

Plus, it's also important to know that mental health medication is different for individuals. It may be possible that your friend is suffering from the same disorder as you. Still, a physiatrist will prescribe various treatments to both of you. The treatment depends upon your personality, symptoms, experiences, and well-being.

Getting better through the use of medication for mental health is a long process. In my case, it took me three years to heal from my traumas. In these years, my doctor prescribed multiple medications to analyze which one is the most effective with minimal side effects. After these three years, I have a medical plan to enhance my quality of life.

In your case, treatment can take many forms, with medication playing a role alongside other therapies such as talking therapies (e.g., cognitive behavioral therapy (CBT)), self-help (e.g., lifestyle changes, guided self-help or physical activity), and alternative therapies (e.g., mindfulness or acupuncture).

According to the National Center for Health Statistics (NCHS), the percentage of adults seeking mental health treatment rose from 19.2% to 21.6% between 2019 and 2021[13]. If nothing else, this statistic proves one thing: you are not alone.

---

[13] https://www.cdc.gov/nchs/products/databriefs/db444.htm

From being the person who used to live in delusions, I am now writing a book that made me revisit the worst times of my life, shedding light on a very sensitive issue—mental health. I want you to be full of hope and remember that if Amber can do it, then why can't you?

My healing journey owes its success to a team of extraordinary individuals, starting with Dr. Troggio, my psychiatrist, who first diagnosed my bipolar disorder. Something I had long mistaken for severe mood swings.

He guided me to confront my "ugly self," urging me to reflect on my past decisions, the people I encountered, the highs and lows of life, and the precious moments with my daughter. His carefully tailored combination of medications brought my symptoms down to zero, laying the foundation for my recovery.

He suggested China Doll Cocktail therapy to me, which was a combination of medication, therapy, involvement of my family members, and spirituality. Fortunately, this therapy worked wonders for me and turned out to be the most effective.

Then, Tynesha White, my second therapist, transformed my perspective. She helped me see myself not as a monster but as a strong, rare, and beautiful 'Black Diamond.'

Throughout this journey, my daughter was my strength and inspiration. She actively participated in my therapy sessions. Her love and dedication fueled my determination to reclaim my life. I am blessed with her.

She taught me that mental disorders are not the problem; neglecting them is.

I'm deeply grateful to both of them—they gave me my life back.

But this chapter doesn't end here. There's something important I need to share.

As I mentioned earlier, recovery from mental illness takes time. Imagine you've started medication, and it's working. You feel great, and you even start thinking that you don't need this anymore to live your life.

That's amazing progress!

But here's the crucial part: your next step should always be consulting your doctor. Stopping medication without their guidance is a dangerous mistake—it can lead to severe setbacks or worse.

I know this because I made that mistake.

I thought I was fine. I stopped my medication without informing Dr. Troggio. I started drinking and smoking again, thinking everything would stay under control.

It didn't.

Within months, I was hit by two massive manic episodes. I was at my lowest point again.

It was my mother who insisted I return to Dr. Troggio. I apologized, and he adjusted my treatment. That day, I promised myself something: I would never stop taking medication without his approval again.

Neither should you.

We must accept that we're not the experts here. Making decisions about medication without a doctor's input can lead to devastating consequences—even death. Let's respect the process, trust our doctors, and take care of ourselves the right way.

IX

And Then Comes 'That Someone'

"True strength isn't found in standing alone—it's discovered in the connections that help you rise, heal, and grow."

-        Amber Rae Johnson Diaz

For years, I thought being independent meant handling everything alone. But this mindset only left me feeling stuck and isolated.

Things changed when I started reaching out to others. At first, I was hesitant. Over time, I became braver and discovered how much strength comes from leaning on people you trust. Not entirely depending upon them and associating your happiness with them but knowing there's someone out there who can help when needed. A ray of light in the darkness, asking for help in times of need.

Support is not just about sharing your problems. It's about building connections that help you move forward.

A friend who listens, a mentor who encourages you, or a professional who offers guidance—all of them play an important part.

Together, these people become your support system. They help you heal, grow, and face life's challenges, no matter how tough they seem.

A support system is a network of people who stand by your side during life's most difficult moments. They provide emotional, mental, and sometimes physical support to help you fight challenges and stand firmly in the face of adversities.

Whether it's friends, family, mentors, or professionals, a strong support system gives you a safe space to share your struggles without fear of judgment.

Healing from trauma is rarely a solo journey. When you feel broken or overwhelmed, the people who love you remind you of your strength. They hold you accountable for showing up for yourself.

It's not just about fixing the pieces. It is about creating a space where you can feel seen, heard, and understood.

For me, building a support system became the turning point in my healing journey. After years of carrying the weight of childhood trauma, broken relationships, and mental health struggles, I realized something important.

Healing required more than just my own efforts.

My support system did not just appear overnight. It was a network I carefully built over time. It was made up of people who truly understood me and my struggles.

Dr. Troggio, my psychiatrist, became one of the first pillars of support. He worked tirelessly to find the right medication to stabilize my bipolar disorder. Alongside him, my therapist, Tynesha White, helped me reframe how I saw myself.

My mentors, like Arlin Lido, played another critical role. Arlin believed in me when the world turned its back on me. She encouraged me to take breaks when needed. I refer to my mentors, family, and friends as my "angels."

Each one has been tied to my journey. They offer guidance, accountability, and unconditional love.

The next important thing I do to heal myself is to surround myself with accountability partners. They are a crucial part of a support system. They help me stay committed to my healing and growth.

Their role is to hold you responsible for the promises you make to yourself. This includes checking in on your progress, encouraging you when challenges arise, and offering honest feedback when needed.

What makes accountability partners so effective is their ability to provide structure. They offer consistency, which is key in a healing journey. When you are overwhelmed, they help you prioritize what matters most. They remind you of your goals and encourage you to keep taking small steps.

For me, accountability partners played a key role in my healing journey.

The most important lesson accountability partners taught me is that healing is not linear. You will have setbacks. You will stumble. But having someone by your side to lift you up and remind you of your strength can make all the difference.

Surrounding yourself with people who hold you accountable creates a space where you can heal, grow, and thrive. And when the worst life experiences like heartbreak shatter you from the core, they will be there for you. Heartbreaks often serve as a catalyst; either they can make you the best version of yourself, or they can tear you into pieces. The choice is yours.

For me, the people I trusted the most became the reason behind my heartbreak. One of my most painful breakups was with Shira, someone who once made me feel safe and cared for. However, when my struggles with bipolar disorder became overwhelming, Shira felt unprepared to support me through it. The relationship ended, leaving me heartbroken and questioning my worth.

It was a tough time, but that's when Austin entered my life. He was a friend and a reminder that there was still good in the world. Austin had a way of making me see things from a fresh perspective. He helped me believe that even after painful endings, there could be new beginnings.

Through our friendship, I learned to open up again. Austin encouraged me to be vulnerable, something I had been afraid of for so long. He showed me that it was okay to let my guard down and trust people, even after everything I had been through. Slowly, I started to feel like I could breathe again.

With the support of a friend like Austin, I began to accept who I truly was. I didn't need to hide behind walls or wear masks. I could be my authentic self, with all my scars and flaws, and still be worthy of love and respect. Austin's friendship reminded me that healing is not about being perfect. It's about accepting yourself as you are and allowing yourself to grow.

As I healed, I also began to reconnect with my faith. Austin shared his own journey of faith with me, and I started to see God in a new light. I realized that God didn't abandon me during my darkest times. Instead, He was there, waiting for me to open my heart again. Our friendship helped me rediscover my connection to God, and through that, I found peace.

What I've learned from my friendship with Austin is that the end of one chapter doesn't mean the end of everything. It's an opportunity to find new strength, discover parts of yourself you may have hidden away, and embrace the journey ahead. Even in the hardest times, there are people who will help you find your way. There is always room for growth, healing, and new beginnings.

If you're facing an ending in your life, whether it's a relationship, a job, or a dream, remember this: it's not the end of your story. It's a chance for you to rediscover who you are and step into the person you were always meant to be.

The right people will come into your life to help you heal and grow, just like Austin did for me.

Life does not end with heartbreak. It is a chapter, not the whole story. My journey is proof that you can rise stronger and wiser. By choosing growth, you allow yourself to step into a new season of life—one filled with hope, purpose, and love for yourself.

If you are struggling with a painful past, remember this: Life is so beautiful. Your heartbreak does not define you. It can be the very thing that leads you to rediscover your strength and create a future you truly deserve.

Take a deep breath, and know that the best is yet to come.

X

A Comprehensive Approach Is What It Takes

"Healing is about blending multiple solutions, not finding one. Approaching problems from all angles leads to true recovery."

- Amber Rae Johnson Diaz

When I look back on my healing journey, it feels like a puzzle that finally came together. At the time, I didn't realize I was combining different approaches and techniques to heal the deepest scars on my soul. The scars I never wanted to share with anyone, the scars I am afraid to open up about in front of anyone.

I was hopeless, broken, and not expecting anything good out of my life. It was fate that directed me toward BDSM at first. It was not like I was well aware of this concept from the beginning. It was new to me; all of it seemed like an 'alien concept' at first. Unconsciously, this concept fell upon me, and eventually, it led me toward my better version, along with medication, therapy, self-care, and spirituality.

This mix became the foundation of my recovery and taught me a very important lesson in my life: "Healing isn't about finding one solution; it's about blending what works for you."

For a long time, I thought medication would make me weak or dependent. I couldn't have been more wrong. Medicine helped calm the chaos in my mind, allowing me to think clearly for the first time in years. My psychiatrist, Dr. Troggio, tailored a plan that seamlessly addressed my symptoms. He reminded me that medication isn't the whole answer, but it's a critical piece of the puzzle. I cannot agree more.

Therapy, on the other hand, taught me how to rebuild my life. My therapist, Tynesha White, helped me see myself not as broken but as someone rare and resilient. She called me a black diamond, strong and unique. Through therapy, I faced my past, learned to forgive myself, and began creating a life that felt worth living.

As I moved forward in my healing journey, I adopted self-care. It may sound simple, but it's often the hardest step to take. For years, I ignored my needs. I thought rest was synonymous with laziness, and saying no was selfish. Slowly and gradually, I learned that self-care isn't about indulgence; it's about survival.

I started small. I wrote in my journal, walked in the sun, and set boundaries in relationships that drained me. These little acts gave me strength. They reminded me that I mattered. When you prioritize your well-being, you're helping yourself.

Thanks to my best friend, Austin, who introduced me to spirituality. It became my anchor when everything else felt uncertain. It wasn't about religion alone but about finding a connection to something bigger than myself. For me, that meant surrendering my pain and fears to God. It was a relief to know I didn't have to carry everything on my own.

After experimenting with multiple things and finally cracking the code to my healing therapy, I am still sticking to my MANTRA that healing isn't a one-size-fits-all process. What worked for me might not work for you, and that's okay.

The beauty of healing is that it's personal. It's about finding the right balance for yourself. The reason why I am sharing my journey with you is not to push you into following my footsteps but to let yourself free and open up to the different methodologies that can lead you to the best version of yourself.

If there's one thing I want you to take away from my story, it's this: healing is possible. It's not easy, and it's not quick, but it's worth it. I'm living proof that you can move from pain to purpose, from surviving to thriving.

Your journey will look different from mine, and that's the way it should be. But know this: you're not alone. There's a path to wholeness waiting for you. Take it one step at a time, and trust that brighter days are ahead.

As I was penning down these words, my eyes were filled with tears. I couldn't believe I had done this. Trust me; this feeling of living for yourself and improving continuously is out of this world. In the middle of the draft, an idea kicked me in, which helped me find a comprehensive approach to healing. I was not a specialist to figure everything out on my own.

What was that hidden superpower of mine? After brainstorming for hours, I found the answer. It was my open-mindedness towards unheard things and unique ideas. In simple terms, it was my multifaced approach to solving any problem.

What If I rejected the idea of BDSM as a whole only because I knew this term only as 'sexual practice'? Perhaps I would have never been able to heal and be able to write this book.

And now, at this point, you should also understand the importance of a multifaced approach to solving any problem.

In life, we all face challenges either big or small. What matters is how we approach the problem or a challenge when we stand right in its face. Some of us take the simple route, looking for a quick solution. But the truth is that most problems are complex and require a multifaceted approach.

They can't be solved with a one-dimensional approach. To find the best solutions, we need to look at things from multiple perspectives.

Multifaceted problem-solving means looking at a challenge from different angles. It's like looking at a puzzle from all sides before you try to put it together. When we approach problems this way, we uncover more solutions and possibilities.

If I had approached my healing journey from just one perspective—only focusing on the medication or only focusing on therapy—I wouldn't have made the progress I did. I needed to consider my mental health, my emotions, my environment, and my lifestyle as part of the solution.

When we approach a problem with a narrow focus, we often miss key details. We might make assumptions, rush decisions, or overlook solutions that could have worked better. A narrow approach doesn't allow us to fully understand a situation, which can lead to more frustration or failure.

For example, when I was first diagnosed with bipolar disorder and PTSD, I only focused on my symptoms. I thought if I just managed the symptoms, I'd be fine. But I soon realized that to truly heal, I needed to consider other factors like my emotional health, my relationships, and my lifestyle choices.

Albert Einstein once said,

"We cannot solve our problems with the same thinking we used when we created them."

Steve Jobs believed,

"Innovation is saying no to a thousand things."

When tackling any problem, it's essential to consider several perspectives to ensure a well-rounded solution. Let's look at some of the perspectives that can help in problem-solving:

Emotional Perspective: Your emotions play a key role in how you view a problem. Be honest with yourself about how you feel. Are fear, anger, or stress clouding your judgment?

Logical Perspective: Sometimes, emotions can get in the way of clear thinking. Logical problem-solving involves looking at the facts. What are the underlying issues causing the problem? What do you need to do to fix them step by step?

Practical Perspective: Ask yourself: what are the practical steps you can take to solve the problem? What resources are available to you? What is realistically achievable?

Long-Term Perspective: Consider how your decisions will affect your future. Will the solution you choose lead to long-term benefits? Will it bring lasting peace or healing? Looking ahead is critical to making sustainable choices.

You may feel confused after having so much at once, though it's not. Let me simplify the concept of solving a problem through multifaced approaches to the most difficult decision of our life: Selecting a Life Partner.

Future Perspective: When choosing a life partner, it's crucial to think beyond the present moment. Will this person share your long-term goals? Can they grow with you as you evolve over the years?

<u>Result:</u> A future-oriented view helps you see whether this relationship will withstand the test of time.

Societal Perspective: Relationships are also influenced by societal pressures and norms. Consider how family, culture, and friends might view the partnership.

<u>Result:</u> While it's important to stay true to yourself, understanding these influences can help you navigate potential challenges in the relationship.

Emotional Perspective: Love and emotional connection are vital. However, it's essential not to let emotions cloud your judgment. A strong emotional bond should be built on respect, shared values, and understanding, not just intense attraction or temporary feelings.

Practical Perspective: It's also important to evaluate practical factors such as financial stability, communication styles, and conflict resolution. Can you both handle disagreements constructively? Do you have complementary lifestyles?

<u>Result:</u> These are essential questions to ask when thinking about the long-term viability of the relationship.

Solving problems from multiple perspectives allows us to find solutions that are well thought out, balanced, and more likely to succeed in the long term.

Whether you're choosing a life partner or selecting a career path, it's important to approach these decisions with a full understanding of all the factors at play. By keeping a diverse set of perspectives in mind, you give yourself the best chance to make choices that truly serve your needs and goals.

The key here is to never give up on yourself.

XI

May I Get The Directions to Peace?

"True peace begins when you take responsibility, embrace your journey, and light the way for others."

-        Amber Rae Johnson Diaz

Have you ever reflected on your day and productivity before going to bed? What's your usual answer? Do you feel content, or do you wrestle with regret and frustration?

For years, nearly 15 to be exact, I went to bed feeling regretful, sometimes even with tears in my eyes. I often asked myself, "What's wrong with me? Why do I struggle with things that seem effortless for others? Am I not good enough?" The questions haunted me.

Countless times, I argued with God (something I'm not proud of). Over time, I realized one significant truth: I had spent years blaming others and external circumstances for everything wrong in my life. This habit started in childhood, and while it may have made sense back then, it grew into a pattern that slowly killed me inside. I never took responsibility for anything, good or bad. I wasn't steering my own life; I had handed over control to the environment around me.

To cut a long story short, I was aimless, unaccountable, and disconnected from any sense of purpose. Days blurred into months and months into years. Then, one day, I decided enough was enough. I gave myself three simple, achievable tasks: limiting screen time to 4 hours per day, doing hair care, and eating healthy. To my surprise, I did. That night, I slept peacefully for the first time in years.

From that moment, I began cracking the code to live a purposeful day, week, month, and year. I started taking my life seriously. What followed were three transformative years, years that rewrote the script of my life. During this time, I experienced a rollercoaster of emotions: love, friendship, hate, and more. I saw incredible highs and crushing lows.

Now, having overcome those challenges, I want to share a concept with you, the "Island of Peace." Don't worry. It's not a physical place, although it could be. The Island of Peace is a mental and emotional state where you live with purpose. You wake up with the intention of doing something meaningful and end the day with most of your goals accomplished. For me, this often looks like giving my daughter a goodnight kiss and going to bed with peace in my heart.

Life isn't a fairytale, nor is it impossibly difficult. Discipline is hard, but the rewards it brings are beyond imagination. My favorite outcome of discipline? Peace is the kind that brings tears of joy, not regret.

The Island of Peace is simple to understand but challenging to achieve. It's about maximizing your potential, mentally and physically. It's about recognizing your strengths, accepting your flaws, and using your unique abilities to fuel your growth. Here's how you can start:

- Identify what's holding you back.
- Pinpoint what you're naturally good at.
- Acknowledge your struggles.
- Discover what you can do for hours without boredom.

Your path to the Island of Peace lies in these answers. This isn't just philosophy—it's a process I've practiced and refined. Believe me, it works.

You're capable. You're worthy. Stop procrastinating and giving yourself excuses. Deep down, you know you can't lie to yourself. Take the first step. Yes, it will be messy at first, but it will lead to blessings.

Whenever I feel like giving up, I simply look at the texts on my wall:

Steve Jobs

"Your work is going to fill a large part of your life, and the only way to be truly satisfied is to do what you believe is great work. And the only way to do great work is to love what you do."

J.K. Rowling

"It is our choices, Harry, that show what we truly are, far more than our abilities."

Emma Watson

"Don't feel stupid if you don't like what everyone else pretends to love. Find what makes you truly happy and fulfilled."

Jim Carrey

"You can fail at what you don't want, so you might as well take a chance on doing what you love."

These quotations not only fuel me but also give me the strength to think big and achieve big.

Let's clear up a common misconception: a productive life isn't about perfection. There's no such thing as a perfect life; perfection is a myth. In my 30+ years, I've never met anyone who flawlessly follows an Instagram-worthy routine. Influencers often sell us beautiful lies, and we fall for them. But we need to stop.

True productivity means ticking off most of your to-do list and striving to improve each day. It's that simple. Yet, we overcomplicate it, set unrealistic goals, and then feel bad when we fail. That's the problem.

If you reduced your TikTok time from six hours last week to five this week, congratulations—you've made progress. Bad habits take time to form, and they take time to break. Work step by step. Reduce gradually and celebrate each milestone.

For me, my Island of Peace is tied to a dream: transforming my grandparents' property into a spa resort for people with bipolar disorder and mental health challenges. This spa would be a judgment-free haven offering mindfulness, self-care, spiritual practices, and even unconventional therapies. Patients would have access to whatever they need, and my sole purpose would be to help them heal.

I refuse to let my 15 years of struggles go to waste. I want my daughter to be proud of me.

I am still learning about myself and growing. I am loving the woman I am becoming. This peace gives me the strength to keep moving forward.

My personal life is important for peace. Faith is a big part of my Island of Peace. I want to share my story to help others. I also hope to inspire people to help others. My main vision of creating a spa is that I want to reach the broken hearts and tired souls that are often forgotten. I believe that a healthy mind is a fuel to growth.

Lastly, I want to feel like a normal person with my unique capabilities. My island of peace is also a process of thriving and growing every single day. I want to be the light in people's dark life.

Author's Note

Alas, we've reached the final chapter. Our journey is coming to a close, and I find it hard to believe.

I'm filled with mixed emotions—happiness, fulfillment, and a sense of loss. It feels as though we've built a strong connection through these pages and words. Before I wrote this book, I had never imagined that something so simple could hold such power to help others.

As you've made it this far, I want you to understand that, consciously and unconsciously, you've reached the most important milestone of my life. It's not just because you've read my story. It's because you chose to prioritize your mental health over everything else.
And for that, I'm incredibly proud of you.

Take a moment to pat yourself on the back for embracing a topic that many shy away from. You've learned and unlearned countless mental health practices alongside me.

Remember: If I can transform from a fragile China doll into a Black Diamond, if I can overcome multiple mental disorders and share my journey.
Why can't you?
What's stopping you?

We've learned that vulnerability is strength. We've learned that having mental health challenges doesn't equate to weakness. And we've learned that surrender is a choice.

Haven't we?

Yes, we have.

Now, all you have to do is start practicing what resonates with you.
What fits your situation, and what brings out the best version of yourself?

I'm not exaggerating when I say this wasn't about money. Yes, money is a powerful asset, but there are things far more powerful than it—one of them is the impact we make.

I want each of you to feel valued, worthy of love, and capable of achieving great things.

I want you to take ownership of your life.
I want you to embrace living with your mental health condition.

And most of all,
I want you to reach the pinnacle of human potential.

I believe in you.

And you must believe in yourself, too.

Stay blessed,
~Amber